DED

First, I would like to say "thank you" to the Lord for the abundant favor that He has placed upon my life. It's is only in Him and through Him that I am able to accomplish anything in this life.

To my wife, I'm eternally grateful for the way you extend so much grace and patience with the many hours I work and am away. I couldn't do this without your love, sacrifice and support. I want you to know that I see you and though I may not say it often enough, I know how hard you work to help me accomplish all that God has called me to do all the while working full-time yourself and being an amazing wife and mother. Without you, I wouldn't be half of the man than I am today.

To the numerous clients who have motivated, trusted and believed in me, you have challenged me in ways I couldn't have grown without and that means more to me than mere words could ever express. This book wouldn't exist if it weren't for each and every one of you.

I also dedicate this to the dreamers. The visionaries. The ones who have a dream but have lost hope of ever making it a reality. If I can do it, so can you! Write the vision and make it plain, create a plan and put a date on it. Then, get started!

Lastly, to everyone who came together to help make this dream a reality, I extend a heartfelt thank you and pray that God blesses you abundantly.

BREAK-THRU

CONTENTS

It was 2011, in the beat up little gym underneath the basketball court of Eastern Connecticut State University. I'm standing in front of a 45 pound bar with weights stacked on each end, and beside me I hear "Let's go, pick it up, you can do it!" That's when it all started, my passion for working out and living a healthy lifestyle was ignited.

When I first met Shane, I was one of those people that would go to the gym and exercise every now and then, mainly when I got to the point where I realized I hadn't been in a while. So, I figured I should probably go just to be able to say "I worked out this week". When I did make it to the gym, because I had absolutely no clue what I was doing, I'd head straight for the treadmill (or elliptical if I wanted to mix it up) and I'd spend the next 15-20 minutes doing some sort of weird jog-run-walk combination while trying to formulate a semi-okay workout plan that would give me sexy abs and a toned booty. Of course, I'd never even consider anything that required me lifting weight with my arms. There was no way I wanted to get "manly, bulky" biceps. So after a few sets of sit-ups and squats, sprinkled with intermittent resting periods to check my text messages, I'd call it a day. If I made it to the 1 hour mark, I'd feel especially accomplished and maybe even make a post on social media about my great workout session and my plans to come back the next day. However, because I really hated the feeling I got from walking around amongst the machines looking like a lost puppy, I probably wouldn't be back for a while. Then, due to lack of motivation to exercise, I also couldn't seem to justify trying to eat healthy. This was me. I had the desire to live a healthy lifestyle, but I had no idea how to do it.

Shane and I started working out together my sophomore year of college. His drive and his motivation to keep going and keep reaching new goals was inspiring to me. He showed me what it was to be strong and to be fit. He trained me and showed me that I had everything I needed right inside of me, I simply needed guidance, direction, and an encouraging push. I wish there was a book like this that was out back then. The way Shane breaks down health and fitness in this book makes it super simple to understand. So much so that all who read it should feel fully equipped to get started on their health and fitness journey. Or maybe, like me, equipped to re-start your journey in a way that will set you up for success.

Now, some may think I'm biased because I'm blessed enough to be able to call Shane my husband. What I WILL say, is this. I have never met a more dedicated, hard worker in my entire life. When I met him 7 years ago, he was an athlete competing with some of the top CrossFit competitors in our region, and he was training others for free just because he enjoyed it. That same drive and zeal that he had back then has only multiplied, and he continues to fan the flame each day when his feet hit the ground. He had a dream to own his own gym, he chased it and he achieved it. He's earned certification after certification, striving to be the best trainer that he can be for his clients. He's dedicated countless hours to making his business better. If you ask him what his business hours are, he'll tell you "From when I wake up, until I go to sleep." There is no one out there who can account for his hard work and dedication the way that I can. No personal trainer I have ever met truly cares about his clients the way that Shane does. He goes above and beyond the call of duty. Whatever their needs are whether it be, finances, time, mental, or spiritual, he meets them.

In Shane's words, he's a hustler. He never gives up. When he told me he was writing a book I thought to myself, "God, you sure do work in mysterious ways. He's constantly moving, and now he's got a book to write on top of it all." Then two days later, the first draft was formed and I had the pleasure of being the first to read it. I am blown away by the content in this book. May it bless and encourage everyone who reads it looking to improve their life, and the lives of those around them.

Ashley Vega

VegaFit Elite Fitness and Training LLC

CHAPTER ONE
The Results Start When You Do

W hen it comes to our bodies, we all want the fastest results and if we are honest, we have gone through some pretty desperate measures to achieve those results. The truth is that deep inside we all know that there are no lasting quick results or easy shortcuts. The "quick results" fads are nothing but attempts to bandage what *really* needs to be dealt with in order to achieve a lifelong, sustained outcome. Quick results never last and can leave you worse off than when you started.

Maybe you're someone who doesn't know where to start and that's okay. We will address that in the next few chapters. First, let's take a look at the necessary steps.

In goal setting, I use the "SMART" goals approach. The acronym S.M.A.R.T. stands for

Specific, **M**easurable, **A**ttainable, **R**elevant, and **T**imely.

1. **Specific -** A generic goal would look something like this: "I want to lose weight, trim my arms, tone my butt, and have abs." A *specific* goal will look more like this: "I want to lose 5lbs in one month; lose 1 inch around my arms; drop 1 pant size; drop down to 15% body fat."

2. **Measurable –** Identify what it is you will see, hear and feel when you reach your goal. Being excited or feeling good cannot be considered measurable evidence that you are meeting your goals. A measurable goal is something you can check each week until the goal is met. For example, body weight or body fat percentage. If a goal of yours is to have more energy, you need to have a way to measure what you consider to be "more" energy, such as feeling alert at 5 p.m. rather than groggy.

3. **Attainable** - Is your goal attainable? This means that your goal is achievable. Do you have the time, money, and talent to reach your goal? Investigate if what you're about to do will be a priority or impede priorities. I see so many clients sign up for training and show up for 2 weeks and then they quit. It's not because they don't want to work out; it's because they didn't think about the "attainability." Their work schedule was interfering; they had poor time management, always hit traffic or they didn't realize how much extra work it would be on top of their regular daily responsibilities.

4. **Relevant** – Is reaching your goal relevant to you? Instead of vague resolutions you need to set a clear milestone so that you don't feel defeated. Important questions to ask yourself are: What is your aim? How will achieving your goal impact your life? What is your "why" or your main motivation? Answering these questions

will give you a deeper connection to your goal and help to keep you motivated.

5. **Timely -** Setting a timeline is key to your success because you don't want to go through life without any accountability to time. Set the time frame in which you want to reach your goals and then check your progress regularly. We all need deadlines, in fact, almost everything we accomplish or are told to so in life whether it be at work or at school, has a deadline. Knowing your deadline will keep you focused and on target.

I have often thought about how often people sign up for an inexpensive gym membership and never go but continue to make regular payments. Why is that? Because those big, inexpensive gyms know that most of their members will not show up 90% of the time. They know that the psychology behind people joining gyms is mostly so that they can *feel* better. They know that the majority really don't mind paying a small fee every month for a gym membership that they'll never use in exchange for the small subconscious payoff of being able to say that they have one.

Now that we have defined the S.M.A.R.T goals, we have to lay the foundation that will be the springboard for these goals. That foundation is knowledge. Get informed! I recommend getting professional guidance from a certified trainer to learn about the right tools for YOU to accomplish your goals. Knowledge is power. We have to know what's realistic and what isn't and a trained professional will be able to help you with that and guide you in the right direction. Tragically, I see too many people who receive advice from someone who isn't qualified, only to end up right back in the same situation they started in or worse. Just because someone is in shape doesn't mean that they know how to teach someone else how to get there. The same method that worked for that person might not be what will work for you.   I am not saying that just because they are not a professional that they are unable to help, but what I am saying is that it's not much different than when you go to a doctor. Just as you don't want someone who's never been to medical school diagnosing your illness, you don't want someone who doesn't know about the body telling you how to get healthy.

As we close the first chapter, I encourage you to take some time to really focus on what you just read and let it sink in. Start thinking about your goals and referring to the list below, write some of those goals out.

Choose two and start here:

- Run 1 mile a week
- Walk 3 Miles a week
- Lose 5lbs in 1 month
- Lose 10lbs in 1 month
- Drop 1 pants size in 3 months
- 30 mins of strength conditioning a day
- Start a meal plan
- Hire a trainer

You can get started here right now and then keep on reading.

My Goals

_____

_____

_____

_____

_____

_____

_____

CHAPTER TWO
Styles of Training

A re you in the right zone? To start with, let's define what I mean by "right zone". I can guarantee that almost everyone has trained in the wrong category at some point and you will learn something from this chapter. If you have never exercised, then this is great for you! You get to skip some of the most common mistakes and do it right the first time. The most common styles of training I would like to stick with are muscular endurance, hypertrophy, strength training, and power training. When we understand these types of training, we can then be effective and efficient in the gym. My studies with the National Academy Of Sports Medicine (NASM) has helped me understand the differences and how they work.

Muscular endurance is the ability to exert force over long periods of time, or, doing high repetitions. (A repetition or "Rep" is one complete movement of a single exercise.) Muscular endurance training is important to increase your stabilization, core, joint strength, power, and muscle building. In time, we must all do muscular endurance exercises to increase the areas stated above. If you are a beginner or are just getting back into the gym, I recommend starting with muscular endurance training. This will help you build a solid foundation.

For example: Muscle endurance training would be 2 sets of 12-20 repetitions. (A set is a group of consecutive repetitions.) Numerous sets and high repetitions will decrease body fat and increase lean body mass.

Muscular Endurance	Reps	Sets	Rest	Frequency	Duration	Exercises
Resistance Training	12-20	1-3	0-90s	2-4/wk.	4-6wk	1-3

When I train clients who want weight loss, I am almost always doing multiple sets for high reps, and that also means lower weight. I have heard clients say "15-20 reps?! What??" It sounds like a lot, just remember high reps + heart rate up = burning fat. For beginners, this phase of training is key to your success before you jump into any other style because you want to increase your core and joint stabilization, strength, and power. It's very much like building a house. Before you build a house, you must have a solid foundation in order for the house to be stable. It's one of the safest ways to work out before moving on to any other style of training to avoid muscle imbalances and injury.

Hypertrophy training seems to be the most popular style of training in today's gyms. Have you ever walked into a gym and seen big guys just staring at themselves in the mirror with their cut off shirts? They are more than likely wanting their muscles to get bigger. Throughout the years I have asked people what they are doing for their workouts, what their goals were, and almost every time they describe hypertrophy training and don't even realize it. They are doing something opposite to what their goal is! When you think of hypertrophy, I want you to think about bodybuilding. Do you want to make your muscles bigger? Hypertrophy training for both men and women who do not exercise often will take about 4 to 8 weeks before they see any results.

The typical rep and set range looks something like this:

Ex. 3 sets of 8-12 reps per exercise or 3 sets of 10 reps

Hypertrophy training requires moderate to heavy weight lifting to see results. Be the judge of what 'heavy' is for you. If you're able to push out every set, you need to move up in weight. Your last 3 reps should be a struggle. Just keep in mind proper form always comes before adding more weight.

If you're twisting, swinging, or jerking the weight please go down in weight (These movements can be performed by experienced lifters.) It is important to perform your exercises slow and controlled. If 8-12 reps in this phase seems too easy, then you need to use more weight. The way I train is to make sure that my last 3 reps feel like they are impossible to accomplish but I push through it!

Hypertrophy Training	Reps	Sets	Rest	Frequency	Duration	Exercises
Resistance	8-12	3-5	0-60s	3-6 times/wk.	4 wk.	2-4 strength exercises per body part.

Maximal Strength training differs from first the two that I have already discussed. You might think, "That's crazy! I thought that was strength training!" When you think of strength training, I want you to think of a powerlifter. Powerlifters are not worried about their size (hypertrophy) but rather strengthening the internal muscles and connective tissue. Powerlifters focus on low reps for max strength.

Have you ever seen the television show "The World's Strongest Man"? On that show they focus on things that test their ability to lift heavy weight in short periods of time. When you bring in the groceries, you may only bring in five bags because you don't have the strength to carry in ten bags. The amount of force in your hand is too much to bear so you can only carry five.

Training for strength focuses on developing maximal strength in individual muscles. In order for you to carry more bags of groceries you have to strengthen your core, grip, forearm, and depending on how you carry your groceries, maybe even your bicep, and your shoulder. Strength training uses low to moderate repetitions with moderate to high volume. (Volume is how many reps or sets you do.)

Strength Training	Reps	Sets	Rest	Frequency	Duration	Exercises
Resistance	1-5	4-6	3-5 min	2-4 times/wk.	4wk	1-3

When you think of power, I want you to think of exercises that involve jumping, throwing, punching, kicking, pulling, and pushing to name a few. Power is producing as much force as you can in the shortest amount of time. You can also use power training with heavy loads to be well rounded in the power-training zone such as doing a clapping push-up with your body weight or with a weighted vest.

So, we must attack power workouts from both sides of the spectrum. We are also working our fast twitch muscles used for powerful bursts. Slow twitch muscles will be for longer distance exercises like running. Power training would be different from doing something slow and steady, to doing something explosive. I can do a back squat slow and then follow it with jumping squats to incorporate strength and power together, creating a superset.

My goal is to give you the simple format and idea of each of these styles of training, not to break down the science behind them. As you move from beginner to intermediate and elite levels, you can increase the number of sets and the number of exercises as you see fit. It is important to train in all of these zones to increase your athleticism, coordination, agility, and overall wellbeing.

Next I want to discuss a variation of resistance training routines you can do to add spice to your workout. I often hear "Shane, I have been working out, eating right, supplementing and it seems like I am not getting any results." What this means is they either are not telling the truth or they may have hit a plateau. A plateau is when you stop seeing changes or breakthrough during your training. Most often, people hit plateaus when there is no variation in their exercise routine, doing the same thing over and over and doing the same exercises on or close to the same days each week. I have been training for 7 years now and muscle confusion is the best way I've been able to get results for both my clients and myself. You should never allow your body to know what is coming. Your muscles have a memory of their own, and they get used to the repetition of the same patterns. I am not saying that a 4 to 6-week routine is bad, what I am saying is most people stay on a routine and never switch it up. I train my clients in a way so they never know what is coming. Every week it's something new and they never have time to adjust because it's varied yet very balanced. That's how I get my clients great results!

With that being said let's look at some variations you can add to your plan:

- **Pyramid** - Increasing or decreasing weight with each set

- **Superset** - Performing two exercises back to back with minimal rest

- **Drop-Sets** - Performing a set to failure, then removing weight and continuing with the set to failure

- **Circuit Training** - Performing a series of exercises, one after the other, with minimal to no rest

- **Peripheral heart action** - Variation of upper and lower body. Performing one upper body workout then one lower body workout.

- **Horizontal Loading** - Performing all sets of an exercise on a body part before moving on to the next body part.

- **Split routine** - Training different body parts on different days.

Do you see how much there is to working out? I am only addressing a few training zones. I suggest spending 4-6 weeks in each zone separately then mixing them together so you are training in all zones and bringing variety into your training.

My clients typically train in a circuit style, which will involve all training zones. However, that is under my supervision and only performed with correct form. I have only named a few of the most popular styles of training, but there are so many ways to train.

However, without the knowledge and understanding of which style of training is for you, you might be wasting your time with your routine. I would rather you be in the gym wasting your time than at home doing nothing. The issue is that some get defeated and discouraged when they don't see the results the're looking for, so I want to help bring that understanding so you can get it right the first time!

What zone of training are you currently in if you are currently exercising? If you are not on a regular exercise routine, muscular endurance would be a great place to start. Here are some routes to take:

- Hire a trainer that can formulate a workout plan personalized for you. It has to be designed for you, your goals, based off your height, weight, age, all these factors are key when designing a workout program.

- Use online resources. There are some good websites out there that provide free starter workout plans.

- If you're not able to punch in your weight, height, and age, understand that these types of templates may not be accurate but will serve as a good enough starting point. Plus, its FREE!

- Join group training in your area. There are always trainers training for free or low cost in large group settings who can help guide you in this area.

You can also do online training so that you can start to get comfortable with the movements to prepare you to do it on your own. I offer training in-person or online at **www.VegaFitElite.com.**

Summary:

Muscular endurance and stabilization is best achieved by performing 12-20 repetitions at 50 to 70% of the one-repetition max.

Hypertrophy (muscle growth) is best achieved using 6-12 repetitions at 75 to 85% of the one rep max.

If maximal strength adaptations are desired, the repetition range is 1-5 at 85 to 100% of the one rep max.

Power adaptation requires 1-10 repetitions at 30-45% of the one rep max or approximately 10% of the body weight.

20 to 30 seconds' rest will allow approx. 50% recovery

40 seconds' rest will allow approx. 75% recovery

60 seconds' rest will allow approx. 85 to 90% recovery

3 minutes' rest will allow approx. 100% recovery

([1]National Academy of Sports Medicine)

My Goals:

_____

_____

_____

_____

_____

_____

_____

CHAPTER THREE
Support System

We all need accountability. It doesn't matter who you are, we all need friends who will provide good accountability to walk this thing out! Even the most elite and professional athletes all have a form of accountability. Workout buddies are great until they bail on you. If you have ever had a workout buddy, you can relate to this. I bet you can't count how many times you asked someone to be your gym partner, and they either came for a short time or got all excited and never showed up. I don't know about you, but that's annoying and discouraging.

There is nothing like having someone there that will push you past what you know you wouldn't have done if they weren't there. It is a great feeling when the workout is completed. Failing workout partners or having someone bail on you and be inconsistent all the time can leave most of us in a downhill spiral. It's hard enough trying to find the motivation as it is, isn't it? That's where personal trainers come into place. I tell my clients if they don't want to train with me anymore that's fine, but I ask they let me help them find another great trainer for them. Trainers are not only the brains of the operation, we are your workout buddy, your friend, your motivator, the person you vent to, the one who has studied hours upon hours, days upon days, months upon months and even years if you have been in the game long enough.

So how do you find a good trainer? I want to give you some things to look for because nowadays licenses and certifications mean nothing. Not meaning to bash new or veteran trainers, (I am speaking to myself as well) but let's be honest, a certification does not give you experience. First, inquire about the trainer; ask how long he or she has been training. This matters because a great trainer also has a wealth of experience. Next, look at the certifications the trainer has earned. Does their certification cater to your needs and the specific goals you are looking for? Don't hire a trainer without knowing their level of experience and certification. That's ignorance! At the same time, this does not mean you should not show new trainers any amount of grace either.

I was there once and I wouldn't be where I am today without the opportunities I received as a beginner. However, use discernment. We know only time can make someone better at what they do and the same applies to their dedication and level of commitment. A dedicated and committed trainer will hold the necessary certifications and will always remain on top of their game with the latest methods based on research and practice. Ask the trainer questions like "What's the toughest client you've ever trained?" "How would you change my work out if I said both my lower back and my knees hurt?" "What are some of your accomplishments?" "Are you pursuing any further education?"

I believe and trust you will have the discernment to wisely judge the answers. You will learn a lot about a trainer based on their responses from your questions. Why am I telling you all of this? Again, because I want you to love this thing called health and fitness! I want you to be as successful as you can be with as little bumps on the road as possible.

First impressions are key when meeting with a trainer for the first time. Listen to your gut. If you and your trainer do not have a connection the first time you meet I would think about looking around until you find someone with a connection. You want to feel comfortable around your trainer always. Of course, in the beginning you might feel a little nervous and that's normal but you shouldn't be questioning them as a trainer. There must be trust! If he or she recommends you do something you should give it a shot. You pay them for their advice and they want to get you results. Their name and reputation are on the line, so I am sure they will give you their best professional advice. They will check up on you, educate you on nutrition, provide you with meal plans, push you beyond your limits, give you their full, undivided attention when you're in a session, and never put you down. A great trainer will provide you with great accountability.

I understand if hiring a trainer is out of the picture due to time and finances. There are other options out there to help you get on your fitness journey. Online training is convenient for people who are always on the go. There are always trainers having free workouts weekly in parks or gyms to market themselves, you just have to look for them online. I am sure I missed some avenues, but the point is that there is no excuse. You can do this with or without a trainer and a workout buddy! The question is, do you want to? If you do, you'll find a way.

Here's the thing about accountability. Many of us say we need accountability but we are not truly allowing anyone to hold us accountable. There is a cost when it comes to having an accountability partner. Relationship is key in order to establish true accountability. Why do

I say that? If you don't have a relationship with that individual, then you won't fully let them in on your weaknesses/struggles. In order to establish true accountability, we must be willing to humble ourselves and accept criticism from that individual. If your accountability partner says to you, "Hey what's going on you missed the gym 3 times this week and were late to every session what's up?" and you get upset at the truth, then you may or may not have a genuine relationship with that person. You could also be dealing with some pride that will block you from moving forward or you may have bitterness towards that person, the list goes on. What I am saying is you must understand that accountability sharpens you. When you see iron sharpening iron, that's a tough process. It isn't gentle and pretty at times but know that you're getting sharper with that individual in your life who is leading you towards taking care of your temple. As iron sharpens iron, so one person sharpens another. Proverbs 27:17

Action:

Make a list of the individuals who you believe will hold you accountable. People who are willing to tell you the truth even though it may hurt. Then sit down with the ones you think are the best fit for you and have a heart to heart. You have to be specific on what that accountability looks like and what you expect from them. This may take some of you out of your comfort zones but I challenge you to take the step of faith and make this personal. A text or phone call will be too shallow. You are looking for true accountability and for them to take this serious. You might even bless them to do the same.

My Goals

_____

_____

_____

_____

_____

_____

_____

_____

_____

_____

_____

_____

CHAPTER FOUR
Nutrition

You feel like what you eat! Oh, boy. This is the part most people don't want to talk about. I get it, you like your soda and snacks that are loaded with sugar. You like grabbing fast food because it tastes good and it's convenient, but let's look at some shocking facts.

Cases of chronic diseases such as cancer, diabetes, asthma and heart disease are on the rise in the United States. According to NASM statistics for 2011-2012, Chronic diseases have become the leading cause of death and disability in the United States accounting for 70% of deaths. 68.6% of adults are overweight or obese. The same trend is happening with our youth ages 2 to 19, with more than nine million overweight. That is staggering! 29.1 million people in the United

States have diabetes, 8.1 million of which may be undiagnosed and unaware of their condition. In adults 20 and older, one in every 10 people suffer from diabetes. Lastly, in those age 65 and older, that figure rises to one in four according to the website diabetes.org.

It's easy to ignore or not see the severity of these statistics until it happens to you or someone close to you. I once told a client who was not taking our training seriously that they were in for a rude awakening. I said "You're going to go to the doctor and they are going to tell you you're in trouble and need to do something fast!" Ouch! I know it sounds harsh, but it was truly out of love because I cared. It hurt me to see them like this. Sadly, a few months later these clients came back to me to let me know that they were suffering from a chronic disease. It is a part of my job to tell my clients the truth, even when it hurts. My client learned a vital lesson, if at first you don't succeed, try doing what your coach told you to do in the first place.

I believe we all have loved ones, people who we care about, who we see living an unhealthy lifestyle. If we truly love them, then we should be having honest conversations offering them support and asking them "how can I help?" People are not born unhealthy or obese, there is always a root to an issue. Many are obese or unhealthy, but hardly anyone cares to ask, encourage, uplift and help people get through it. I understand it may be a crawl, but crawling is better than staying still.

As I said in the opening of this chapter, we are what we eat, so let's talk nutrition for a moment. Check out the word nutrition as defined by the *National Academy of Sports Medicine*. "Nutrition is the process by which a living organism assimilates food and uses it for growth and repair of tissues." We must understand how what we're putting into our bodies affects us. Our bodies are to be fuelled for growth and repair, yet we are putting things into our body that can poison us, cause decay, and can even cause death. Sometimes it's too late to reverse the effects. However, this doesn't have to be the case. We can start today making smarter choices.

Some signs that it's time to change your diet are low energy, difficulty sleeping, constipation, regular headaches, moodiness and even anxiety. Just as there are foods and beverages that will deplete you, there are also tons of food and beverages that will revive you! The change will rock your world and pack a powerful punch.

While I am not a licensed nutritionist, as a personal trainer I do know that nutrition and exercise work together for maximum health. Therefore, I want to go over the fundamentals of nutrition and tell you what to look for so that you can be educated on the basics. Let's get started.

According to NASM, the primary function of protein is to build and repair body tissue and structure. We need to be feeding our bodies protein in order to get the essential amino acids that would otherwise leave our bodies deficient. To make this simple, there are two kinds of amino acids: essential and nonessential. The body can't make essential amino acids so they must come from food sources. I could list all of the essential amino acids for you, but to be honest, most of them only rocket scientists can pronounce. However, you can always look them up if you're interested. I'd much rather focus on keeping this understandable and doable.

If you are a woman, I have some important facts for you to be aware of. I know many of you may hear the word "protein" and immediately think "I don't want to get bulky." Let's throw that myth out right now! The truth is, most women have lower levels of protein compared to men due to their lower caloric intake. Women should actually be taking protein to bring balance to their bodies especially during and after pregnancy which I discuss in the chapter "Baby Weight".

So how much protein should you be taking on a daily basis? NASM recommends if your activity level is sedentary or that of an inactive adult then you will need 0.8 (0.4 g/lb.) grams of protein per kilogram of body weight a day. If you are considered a strength athlete, then you will need 1.2-1.7(0.5-0.8 g/lb.) grams of protein per kilogram of body weight per day, and endurance athletes will need 1.2-1.4 (0.5-0.6 g/lb.) grams of protein per kilogram of body weight. Your protein intake should come from foods such as lean meats, fish, and beans.

Protein supplements should never replace food. In fact, Studies have shown that there is no evidence that proves using protein supplements to replace food is beneficial anyway.

With that said, there are some benefits to **supplemental protein** such as:

- Getting Amino acids before and after your workout
- Aids in weight loss.
- Aiding Athletes who are preparing for competitions and are looking to increase lean muscle mass.

Now, how about that dreaded word CARBS? This might already be going against everything you have believed, but carbohydrates are actually a superior source of energy for the body. Carbohydrates are usually classified as sugars, starches, and fiber. Over the years I have learned that we have something called a **carb flame**. Imagine you have started a fire. You need to constantly add wood to keep the fire burning, right? Well the carb flame is something that responds the very same way when we are doing high intensity workouts. Our body is fuelled by carbs. Runners, for instance, have rehydrate gel packs loaded with carbs. Why? To fuel their carb flame.

Now the reason carbs have a bad reputation is that some people say that it makes you gain weight. Let me break down how this happens. Carbohydrates expand and make you fuller. If your total recommended caloric intake (the amount of calories you should be eating in a day) is 2,000 calories and you have eaten 2,200 calories, what's going to happen?

You're going to exceed your daily caloric intake and store fat in your fat tank. **Fat** is an anatomical term for loose connective tissue composed of cells that store fat called **adypocytes**. Its main role is to store energy in the form of fat. It also cushions and insulates the body. In order to lose weight we need to burn more calories than we are eating, so we need carbohydrates. Carbohydrates are a great source of energy and with that being said, they are there to be burned.

So, you see, the problem carbohydrates, it is simply that we are eating more than we burn, so it is being stored as fat. We are eating unhealthy fats and too much sugar without enough activity. I am not saying go out and eat unhealthy carbohydrate snacks and meals but what I *am* saying that is you shouldn't avoid healthy carbs. I hope this has cleared up some of the confusion surrounding carbs.

The next important term as it pertains to nutrition is called **glycemic index** or GI. The GI of a food has to do with how food affects blood sugar levels, which in turn will help you choose your foods more wisely. There are **high GI** foods and **low GI** foods. Foods with a low GI give sustained energy over a longer period of time, which helps to curb cravings. High GI foods give lots of energy really fast, but cause a quick crash afterwards, which leaves you feeling hungry again. So try to stick to foods with a low GI.

Low foods on the GI chart from lowest to highest would be:

- Peanuts

- Plain Yogurt

- Soy Beans

- Peas

- Cherries

- Barley

- Grapefruit

- Link Sausage

- Black Beans

- Lentils

- Skim Milk

- Fettuccine

- Chickpeas

- Chocolate Milk

- Whole-wheat spaghetti

- Apple

- Pinto Beans

Moderate:

- Apple Juice

- Snickers

- Peach

- Carrots

- Brown Rice

- Strawberry Jam

- Power Bar

- Orange Juice

- Honey

- Pita Bread

- Plain Oatmeal

- Pineapple

- Sweet Potato

- Coca Cola

- Raisins

- Cantaloupe

- Whole-Wheat Bread

High:

- Life Savers

- White Bread

- Bagel

- Watermelon

- Popcorn

- Graham Crackers

- French Fries

- Grape Nuts

- Shredded Wheat

- Gatorade

- Corn Flakes

- Rice Cakes

- Pretzels

- Baked White Potato

- Instant Rice

- Gluten Free Bread

- Dates

This list should be a great starting point for you to begin making healthier food choices.

The last thing I'd like to discuss in this chapter is **dietary fiber**. Fiber is something I believe is not spoken on enough. Fiber is an indigestible carbohydrate. There are two types of dietary fiber, soluble and insoluble. **Soluble fiber** is easily digested by the digestive tract and has many benefits, including moderating blood glucose levels and lowering your cholesterol. Examples of soluble fiber are oatmeal, fruits and veggies.

Insoluble fiber does not digest the same way soluble fiber does. In fact, it passes through the digestive tract close to its original form but offers benefits to intestinal health such as relieving constipation. The recommended fiber intake for young men is 38g per day and 25g per day for women. If you are nowhere close to those numbers then you might find yourself with stomach discomfort, irritable bowel syndrome, or irregularity.

A few common questions in regards to nutrition are:

When should I eat before a workout? One to four hours before a workout is essential so that you are not working out on a full stomach. If you're working out in the morning, this is especially important because **glycogen** (sugar) levels are low. Glycogen is your body's fuel. 80% of your energy comes from glucose and glycogen, so in the morning you are running on fumes until you eat something. I recommend healthy carbs before a workout to regain energy and sustain you during your workout. Some people are unable to eat in the mornings, so a meal replacement could fill that nutritional gap. We need to make sure that we are eating something because we need fuel to burn and get us through the workout. Keep it small and simple. Have you ever felt nauseous or so fatigued during a workout that you thought you were going to vomit?

I see this happen so many times with my clients. In fact, if you're reading this and you have trained with me before, you're probably laughing because you know what I am talking about. Most likely you either did not eat before you worked out, or you had a high GI food that caused your sugar levels to drop. When this happens with my clients I stop to either give them a piece of fruit or a rehydration drink that has carbs, sodium, and low sugar. Within five minutes every time they start to feel better because their sugar levels were low. They were running on fumes! After your workout, you have a 90-minute gap to get protein into your body to stimulate **protein synthesis** (repairing muscle tissue or rebuilding). We want to feed our muscles immediately after our workout. Food takes too long to process in time to get to your muscle so a protein shake is definitely the way to go. The longer you wait the more likely you are to miss the window.

Does eating at night make me gain fat? The answer is NO! Let me explain. If your caloric intake for the day is 2,000 calories and you have only eaten 2 meals for the day, totalling to 1,500 calories, then you eat a meal at night that's 500 calories, you've just reached your 2,000 calories. You have not exceeded your daily caloric intake. You also burned 2,000 calories by the end of your day. So how could you gain fat? The only way you can store fat in your fat tank is by eating more calories than your daily intake is supposed to be. (I recommend that you speak with a trainer or registered dietician to come up with the accurate numbers based off of your goals, if you are able.) So, don't worry about eating at night. Just figure out how much you should be eating in a day and track it. I know that put smiles on lot of people's faces!

Should I be eating fat free foods? One of the first changes people tend to make when they want to incorporate healthier food into their diet is choosing fat free foods, thinking that because it says fat free that it is good for you. I fell victim to this as well. What you might not know is just because it says fat free doesn't mean it's beneficial. Fat free foods can be loaded with carbs and fillers that cause you to gain weight. In actuality you want to be eating healthy fats to flush out the bad fats in your body. Healthy fats can be found in foods such as avocados, fish, almonds, pistachios, nuts, and seeds. Unhealthy fats come from foods like fried chicken, donuts, margarine, and butter. Saturated fats are a definite risk for heart disease and can raise bad cholesterol levels. Unsaturated fats raise good cholesterol levels and can decrease the risk of heart disease. Monounsaturated fatty acids found in olive and canola oils and polyunsaturated fatty acids (found in salmon) are good for the heart and may even prevent cancer, arthritis and hypertension. It's better to choose low fat foods over fat free foods. Therefore, don't just try eliminating all fats, start by adding healthy fats to your diet today.

How much water should I drink? "Babe, have you drank any water today?" I am always asking my wife if she drank her water because I know if she has a headache, is moody, or not feeling well, most of the time it's because she hasn't had enough water. Approximately 60% of the adult human body weight is water. We can only survive a few days without water so this should tell you already how important water is. Sedentary men should consume 3.0L (Approximately 13 cups) and women 2.2L (Approximately 9 cups) of water per day. If your goal is fat loss, you should drink an additional 8 ounces for every 25 pounds above your target weight according to NASM. Water in and waste out. For most individuals, this is a valid statement. If you are drinking four bottles of water a day that's still not enough water. Some of us feel like it's a lot of water because we are not used to reaching our recommended daily allowance but we must strive to reach this goal for our own good. Reaching to hit this goal will change the way you think and most importantly how you feel.

I hope this chapter on nutrition has given some insight on how to tweak your diet concerning some of the most common topics, while eliminating confusion. I based what was addressed in this chapter on the most common questions and concerns I have received over the past few years. My intent is to keep things simple, not to give you the science behind everything. I want this to feel doable to you! Being able to relate creates an image in our minds so that we won't forget the next time we see a label or hear someone talking about nutrition. You will most likely hear these questions or people talking about these topics from here on out, because now you are paying more attention! It's like when you buy a new car you suddenly see it everywhere, right? Keep your ears open you'll see.

Action: Set a goal today to limit some of the junk in your diet. I'm not asking you to remove anything just yet, we're taking baby steps. Simply put aside that bag of chips, soda, candy, whatever it is for you. I am leaving you with a few options to make healthier choices below.

Breakfast:
2 Eggs (Boiled if time is an issue prep the night before)
1 banana
1 Slice of whole grain toast with almond butter

Snacks:
1/2 Cup blueberries
Large Piece of celery with peanut butter
1 Rice cake
1 Chobani yogurt with 1 tablespoon of chia seeds

Lunch:
1 Chicken breast
1 Cup Broccoli
1/2 Cup Brown Rice

Dinner:

Bison burgers
Lamb chops
Sautéed sweet potatoes
Kale and Spinach Salad
Quinoa

Pick up a personalized meal plan at
www.VegaFitElite.com.

My Goals:

_____

_____

_____

_____

_____

_____

_____

CHAPTER FIVE
False Rewards vs Food Satisfaction

I t's more than meets the eye! That's the thought that occurred to me as I contemplated this next chapter. I'm not a psychiatrist or an expert in the area of human thinking by any means, but I'd like to come at you from that angle in a way that perhaps many of you can relate. Let's talk about why we respond the way we do to things we bring into our bodies and why our bodies respond the way they do when we deprive them from certain things.

For the sake of keeping this book easy to read and the contents crisp, I'm only going to touch on the basics. Of course, if you'd like to learn more, you can always go to my website:

There's a common problem that can remain hidden in the dark because it can mask itself as just regular lack of self-control or weak willpower, and that is called **food addiction**. Dictionary.com defines addiction as, "the state of being enslaved to a habit or practice or to something that is psychologically or physically habit-forming." I believe that if we can identify and shine a light on this, it could engage the bomb that blasts the door off of what's standing between those to whom this applies and their breakthrough.

So, let me ask a serious question. Could it be that you have an addiction and don't even know it? Keep reading!

Do you ever wonder why you always feel the need to grab a snack during a movie? Or why you *crave* sugar? Ever ask yourself why you feel good after eating those gummy bears (my favorite) or why the smell of your favorite comfort food mom cooks gives you the warm fuzzies? I'm going to propose that all of this started in your childhood. Anytime we would watch a movie we would eat popcorn, ice cream or whatever was your preferred choice. Mom or dad would reward us with a snack if we behaved or did something good, right? Every time we ate that snack we felt happy. It was almost like a warm hug that remains the same way today. But why is that?

So I did some research to find out at what point we release either **serotonin** or **dopamine** when we eat. Both of these brain chemicals are 'feel good' chemicals. Serotonin releases a sense of calmness, lessens depression, improves your mood, and relaxes you. Dopamine releases a sense of concentration, clarity and alertness. I don't know about you but I feel more clear minded after I eat. Have you ever sat in a meeting or tried to have a conversation with someone and you could not give him or her your full attention because you were so hungry? This chemical release is how our bodies respond to being hungry. If you're an alcoholic, you didn't just wake up and arrive there overnight. An alcoholic drinks regularly for quite some time in order to up a tolerance for alcohol. Well, the same goes for food such as junk food, fast food and sugary food. Eaten regularly, we build a tolerance. That first bottle of Dr. Pepper turns into two, then 3, then 4, then 5 a day. Our bodies build up a tolerance. Then what happens when we try to cut down on those things? The moment we try to cut back, we now begin to deplete the chemicals in those items, hence causing the brain to wonder what is up. That's why it can be such a nightmare to stop drinking coffee, energy drinks and eating certain "comfort" foods. Here come the **withdrawals**!

Withdrawal is the bodies response to a depletion of addictive substances. Our bodies will begin to experience any number of symptoms including but not limited to headaches, anxiety, depression, sweating, shaking, anger, and disorientation. This can last days, weeks or even months. Coffee lovers who have tried to stop can certainly relate!

You try to quite coffee, the headaches kick in and run right back to the coffee to feel better. It was too painful to go through the process of withdrawal, so we go right back attempting to fix the problem with the cause of the problem. It's a never-ending cycle.

In order to end the cycle, we must change our thinking about food. In order to change our thinking about food, we need to ask ourselves some tough questions and be honest with our answers. Do you find yourself unable to control your food intake especially when it comes to sugary junk foods? Do you feel like you "have to have" any certain food or beverage, in order to get through the day? Have you tried numerous fitness and weight loss programs and nothing has worked? Do you feel the need to work out immediately after you eat or find yourself feeling guilty after eating? Many food addicts find themselves trying numerous methods to get healthy. Most of these efforts are focused on ways to lose weight, such as using supplements, programs, drugs, surgery, etc. Some food addicts may even find themselves taking laxatives or purging after they eat to keep the weight off. Do you feel emotional often? Food addicts often feel sad, lonely, hopeless, and embarrassed to eat around people due to their weight. Food addicts will also eat when they are upset and reward themselves with food when they do something good. Do you feel like you battle depression, suicidal thoughts, or often find yourself on an emotional roller-coaster? At gatherings are you more interested in what is being served to eat than you are interested in being around people? Do you often feel preoccupied with being uncomfortable because you do not have proper fitting clothes? Do you steal other people's food? Do you often like to eat in secret? I know these are some intense questions and to some they seem strange to ask, but they are all possible warning signs that there is a greater problem than you originally thought. Food addiction is a serious matter. The first step is acknowledging that there is a problem and then admitting that you need help. Nothing is too big for you to conquer once you pinpoint the problem! I highly recommend that anyone who suspects that they have a real food addiction should seek professional counselling or coaching. It's important to know that you are not alone in this. We all battle to some degree with this, some more than others. You don't have to be obese in order to struggle with food addiction, it can happen to anybody, so don't eliminate or isolate yourself.

Not all food addiction is about food. For me, it was about working out. I was addicted to working out and up until a few years ago, I didn't even know it! Now, before you roll your eyes and say how you'd love to have that problem, hear me out.

Growing up I was always called skinny, scrawny, slim Jim, any word that denotes being "small". Family members would say I had a bird chest (flat chest for a guy), and coming from the people closest to me, I took it very close to heart. It bothered me deeply. Inside, I didn't know this but I had determined that no one would be able to say those things about me again.

My mentality was twisted. If I didn't work out 7 days a week I wasn't a nice person to be around. Of course, I was in denial and masked it well, but my wife didn't enjoy being around me and if you are married you know, that's a serious problem! I would put working out before everything. I cared more about how everyone looked at me physically than I cared about my character. I own my own gym, so I would try to justify my reasons for working out. I allowed myself to believe that in order to fit the role of a personal trainer, I had to keep myself in peak condition.

I began to hate working out and I just did it because I was in a routine. It was no longer enjoyable to me.

I'm not sure what it was specifically, but one day I hit a point where I knew that I needed to get my priorities right. This had gotten way out of control and I had to admit that I had a problem. I needed to discover what the root to my problem was (the hurtful words from when I was a child) and then expose it to someone I could trust. For me, that person was my wife.

To this day my wife will check on me and hold me accountable. Sometimes she will remind me to rest and take a break. Again, there's that word "accountability" again. See why it is so important?

I don't know if someone said something to you to cause you to take the route that you're on today or if they are still affecting you but I'm shining a light on this possibility just in case it exists. There is hope for you. It's important to forgive those whom may have hurt you so that you can be set free and move forward. Also, forgive yourself! Seek wise counsel. You cannot overcome these battles alone. When you start to expose those addictions or wounds you will be surprised how many people around you are battling the same thing.

Action: If you have access to the individuals who hurt you get a hold of them and talk to them. Don't hold on to it. Expose your addictions or strongholds to the people around you so that they can hold you accountable. Seek help from your pastor or trained professional counselor so that he or she can help guide you into being the healthiest you that YOU can be!

Write a list of the people you need to talk to and any emotional issues you wish to conquer this year.

My Goals:

_____

_____

_____

_____

_____

_____

CHAPTER SIX
I Don't Like Taking Supplements

Y ou'll thank yourself when you start to take supplements! Why supplements? Supplementation is used to fill any nutritional gaps, bringing balance to our bodies. I cringe when people say they don't need supplements. The only way you don't need supplements is if you're eating a super strict diet. Very few people obtain all the nutrients they need on a daily basis from food alone, according to Dr. Todd Miller from AdvoCare's Sports Advisory Council. (Dr. Miller has a Ph.D. in Exercise Physiology at Texas A&M, a B.S. of Exercise and Sport Science at Pennsylvania State University and Postdoctoral Training at University of Pennsylvania School of Medicine. He has an amazing YouTube channel with tons of information if you are interested.)

I am not a scientist but I have been studying and teaching people how to live a healthy lifestyle since 2009. If you are skipping meals, not eating fish regularly, drinking soda/energy drinks or fancy coffees (sugar and cream filled coffee) and/or always feel tired, these are clear signs that you are lacking important vitamins and nutrients. Supplements are needed as a healthier alternative. These are just a few examples.

For instance, a **meal replacement shake** will fill in for a missed meal. It's not the preferred replacement for food but it's better than nothing. If you're not getting high-quality **Omega 3's** from a food source, then you should be taking a high-quality fish oil. This is key for brain function, your heart, reducing inflammation, lifting your mood, healthier hair, skin and nails. It also flushes out the bad fats while depositing the good fats.

Essential Vitamins for Men/Women:

* High Quality Multivitamin

* High Quality Fish Oil

* Vitamin D

* Calcium

* Magnesium

* High Quality Protein

When I say high quality, I mean that the vitamin has high potency and is made with safe ingredients. Also, that it's suitable for your age, height, weight, age, level of activity, and your goals. To find out what is right for you contact a trainer or nutritionist.

Nowadays we see supplementation abused all over the place. I think this is why so many people are afraid of it. We see people either taking supplements to get big muscles or to lose a dramatic amount of weight. That's not proper supplementation. If a company is saying "Here drink these shakes and they will replace all your meals" RUN! Nothing can replace food. The best nutrients come from food. What you may not know is that the ingredients in most of the supplements you see are dangerous.

The FDA approves just about anything and puts them on the shelves. Have you heard of the stories of people dying from pre-workout supplements and being rushed to the hospital? Or, the stories of steroids in pre-workout supplements and professional athletes being suspended for testing positive for steroids? I became victim to abusing and using poor quality supplements in college and it began to ruin my already sensitive stomach.

Supplements are not one size fits all and you must have knowledge on how to choose them wisely because new products are coming out all the time.

Have you ever walked into a retail vitamin store, and the moment you walked in the sales associates immediately try to refer you to their store brand product? I am not saying they don't know what they're talking about but why would they only recommend you to their particular brand? Sometimes people don't have your best interest at heart. Be Careful. Do your research on all the ingredients you're putting into your body.

- Some benefits of supplements include but are not limited to:

- Reverses low energy
- Prevents nutritional deficiencies in the elderly
- Prevents chronic diseases or slows the progress of other diseases (Crohn's, digestive disorders)
- Assists in prenatal care for pregnant women who need specific vitamins
- Helps achieve high levels of activity
- Aids in muscle recovery after working out
- Boosts your immune system
- Preps for sport specific training
- Aids in preparing for or after medical procedures such as surgery

Everyone's body reacts differently to different supplements. For instance, I cannot have whey or casein protein. The dairy in the protein does not sit well with my stomach. I prefer more of a plant based protein shake because I can digest it more comfortably. What are the differences between **whey**, **casein**, and **soy** proteins you might ask?

Whey protein is the liquid remaining after milk that has been curdled and strained. It is a byproduct of the manufacture of cheese or casein and has several commercial uses. According to Wikipedia, you can use whey protein to increase your protein intake, for weight loss, or to increase lean muscle mass. Adding whey protein to you diet will keep your metabolism high which will help you burn calories if you're looking for weight loss. Whey protein also contain the **9 essential amino acids**.

We need essential amino acids in our daily diet because our body cannot produce them on their own. There are also **nonessential amino acids** that can be made by the body but we already touched on those earlier. If you have a lack of amino acid in your diet you are at risk of muscle damage, loss and repair. The protein we get from food is broken down into aminos which are used to build and maintain our muscle tissue.

So, what are the 9 essential amino acids?

These are key to remember:

Histidine: For cell replication and very good for children but recent studies show this is good for adults as well.

Isoleucine: Promotes muscle recovery after your workout. Assists with regulating your blood sugar and energy.

Leucine: Stimulates release of insulin from the pancreas and protects your muscles. Leucine deals with tissue healing/skin repair as well as energy production.

Lysine: Prevents herpes infections

Methionine: Breaks down fat, primary source of sulfur in the body. This amino is critical for removing mercury and lead from the body.

Phenylalanine: The body converts this into tyrosine, brain chemicals, L-Dopa, epinephrine, norepinephrine, and thyroid hormones.

Tryptophan: Used to produce serotonin, good for normal brain and nerve functions. This chemical called serotonin is detrimental to sleep, pain control, mood swings, intestinal peristalsis and more.

Valine: Stimulating effects that are needed for muscle metabolism, repair and growth of tissue and maintaining the nitrogen balance in the body.

Casein protein is the name for a family of related phosphoproteins. These proteins are commonly found in mammalian milk, making up 80% of the proteins in cow's milk and between 20% and 45% of the proteins in human milk, according to Wikepedia. Casein digests slow. When I say slow I mean it can take up to 7 hours to digest. What this means is it will sustain you for longer. Some people like to take it before bed so that they know it's at work while they are sleeping.

Soy protein is a protein that is isolated from soybean. It is made from soybean meal that has been dehulled and defatted. Soy protein is known to be plant based and used for weight loss. Due to soy's estrogen like compounds called **isoflavones** this protein usually benefits women more than men. However there has been lots of controversy over this topic.

As you can see, as far as protein goes, there are many to choose from. There are also blends of these proteins together. Can you take more than one kind? Yup. In fact, it wouldn't hurt if you did because each protein breaks down differently and brings something different to the table.

Now if you're someone who just doesn't want to take supplements, I understand. Your diet just needs even more attention. Understand, itt will be difficult and time consuming making it more challenging for you to reach your goals in the amount of time you're probably thinking, without supplements. I have trained more people than I can count and the ones that don't supplement and eat BIG (eat a lot of whole foods to fill in the gaps) move like turtles. They get discouraged quickly and are more likely to give up. Knowing what you are in for won't set you up for failure.

Before I close this chapter I have one more thing to add for all of you seeking a quick boost in your day through beverages. Drinking soda and energy drinks are the equivalent to poison. Coffee isn't horrible but it certainly isn't really beneficial either. Personally, I have my clients supplement these drinks for a healthier drink that is sugar free, has 21 vitamins and minerals, heightens your mental focus and clarity without the jitters, shakes, or crashes. That's a win in my book!

Action: Should you take supplements or shouldn't you? It's ultimately your choice. Here is a list of supplements I recommend because I know that they are safe. You can find these at **VegaFitNutrition.com**. Please be wise and look at the supplemental facts if you have any allergies. You can also email us at shane@vegafitelite.com for any questions or concerns.

I would love to walk you through what might best suit you.

1. MNS 3, C, or E
2. Spark
3. Omegaplex
4. Catalyst
5. Rehydrate

My Goals:

_____

_____

_____

_____

CHAPTER SEVEN
Get Up and Get Moving

Where there is a will, there is a way! How many times have you tried to get into a routine and you stopped because whatever got in the way got the best of you? I want to encourage you not to give up! Let's stop saying we don't have time or the finances to work out when the truth is that we just need to adjust our priorities. How about trying to turn off your cell phone for a half hour, skip that TV show, and stop scrolling up and down social media... c'mon, I know you have some time. If you're always on the go because you travel for business, you have time to get healthy too!

When you are in your hotel room all you need are 20-30 minutes before bed. It's totally doable. You don't even need equipment but if you wanted to, you could pick yourself up some resistance bands to take with you or a DVD to pop in to follow.

If you have kids and you are running crazy all day, that's great! Get them involved in your workout at home. Kids like to stay busy. They follow everything we do, and will do whatever they see you do. Isn't that a beautiful picture? So exercise and they will exercise! In a world where fast food and laziness runs rampant, teaching your kids at a very young age the importance of exercise will give them the advantage that you didn't have!

So can you tell that I'm trying to eliminate just about every excuse we use not to workout? If you find yourself still complaining and trying to figure out why you can't workout, it's because you know that you are in desperate need to but are trying to avoid it. Friend, today I would like to encourage you that you will no longer be stuck in a debate on whether or not to workout. You know who depends on mommy, daddy, or their friend to be healthy and fit? The person sitting right next to you.

I want to speak to the moms for a second or maybe even the stay at home dad. (I am a stay at home dad) I am by no means trying to say I am a mom but I think I could relate in a sense. I have been with my daughter Juliet for almost 3 years as a stay at home dad and man am I tapped out at the end of the day. The first 4 months of her life I seriously did not want to work out. In fact, I hardly did and I lost a lot of weight due to stress (women usually gain weight due to stress). So what got me ticking again? I had to sit down and make a plan.

Most of us don't sit down, make a plan and say "Okay this is where the gap is in my schedule and whether I'm tired or not I'm working out at this time." Without a plan, it's easy to get caught up in our day not realizing there is time. I know that when there is time, you may be too tired to workout for even 30 mins but you have to push through or it's going to get even harder the more you pull away from it.

The more you let your body go, the harder you're going to have to work to get it back. I never thought in my life that I would be able to relate but it was tough! Listen, I am a trainer and I am being real here. My legs were so weak that I was struggling with 95lb squats and for a guy my age that's embarrassing. It hurt, I wanted to puke every time I worked out. I was super discouraged but I kept pressing and you should do the same. I know you can!

C'mon!

This all ties back in to your accountability partner. If you have that lined up and are doing what I am challenging you to do, this step will be significantly easier for you. A great accountability partner will come get your butt off the couch and say let's go, we're working out or even just going on a walk.

Your days might have to start a little earlier or your nights might have to end a little later. Everything worthwhile calls for sacrifice.

What you'll gain is far more valuable than anything you might be giving up.

You don't want to end up being a burden to your family and maybe even your friends one day. Yes, I said burden. God forbid something happens to your health; you're not the only one paying for it. Your whole family takes a hit with either medical bills, stress, it can even cause divorce, you sacrifice not being able to play with your kids (ouch) and the list goes on. I know that's not something you're looking forward to but the time is now. Today. Make sure you're writing down your goals, plans, visions, and get there. As I keep repeating because it's so key, know your WHY.

Action: If you're reading this book you have time to get up and get moving. Start a timer and add up all the time you spend on social media, watching TV, or just playing games. You'll be shocked at how much time you actually have. The excuses stop today! Write down the amount of time you think you spend then actually time yourself. Write down what days/times you'll add exercise to your day and get started now!

Social media time:
Watching TV:
Playing games on my phone or computer:
Talking on the phone:
My Goals:

_____

_____

_____

_____

_____

_____

_____

CHAPTER EIGHT
Baby Weight

Exercise during and after pregnancy, that's the best way to manage baby weight.

Does working out while you're pregnant seem impossible? Do you look at pregnancy as an excuse to eat whatever you want and not have to work out? Ouch! I see this happening all the time, so my goal in this chapter is to address the pre and post baby health and fitness questions that I get asked most often.

According to NASM, there are many benefits for mom and baby from exercising during pregnancy. As a mom, the first thing that you're worried about is safety of the baby, definitely. However, fears that the fetus may be harmed during exercise can be minimized with proper precautions. Women who were previously engaged in exercise before pregnancy may continue with moderate levels of exercise until their third trimester according to NASM.

What type of exercise is moderate? You determine that based off your own level of training, pre-pregnancy. When you see pregnant women training intensely, it is likely that they trained even more intensely pre-pregnancy. I got to see my wife go through this phase first hand.

In the first few months of pregnancy she was fine. She was running, doing deadlifts, planks, and sit-ups. She was engaging in most of the regular exercises she was doing before she was pregnant. Gradually, I began to see her body start reacting to different activities. For example, she could no longer run because she was experiencing cramps. She had to start listening to her body. It was time to slow down and start modifying the workouts. As her stages of pregnancy progressed, the slower and slower she moved. She never stopped working out because she understood the many benefits of exercise during pregnancy.

Core stabilization, flexibility, and strengthening the pelvic floor muscles during pregnancy are important factors to remember during pregnancy. Working on these areas will increasingly work in your favor during delivery. I experienced how important this was when my wife delivered our daughter in three pushes and recovered quickly. Like I said earlier though, she never stopped exercising and strengthening her core. Some things to be careful about are twisting, turning rapidly and performing exercises on your stomach or even on your back. You should be especially careful with these movements in your second and third trimester. During pregnancy, your muscles have more elasticity and can easily be over stretched. Be careful not to over stretch but remember that you should still be stretching as if you weren't pregnant. Whatever you do, no NOT push the limit while pregnant.

Dizziness, nausea, fatigue, shortness of breath, abdominal pain and vomiting are all natural side effects of being pregnant but if any of these occur during exercise you should stop immediately. If you are experiencing any leakage or bleeding after a workout you should contact your health care provider immediately.

If you take the necessary precautions and listen to your body, then you should continue to work out. Trust me when I say you're doing yourself a disservice by not exercising. You should remember that you are no longer one person so you need to amp up the vitamins and minerals you are taking for both you and your baby. Prenatal vitamins have the essential needs that a baby should get for their development pre and post-partum. I recommend whole food prenatal vitamins because they are the best quality. You also want to find yourself a high quality prenatal fish oil with high levels of **DHA** (docosahexaenoic acid) (600mg) and **EPA** (eicosapentaenoic acid) (120mg). This is essential for the baby's brain development.

Studies have shown that babies who received EPA and DHA rather than those who have very low levels of EPA and DHA turned out to have better brain function and are even more intelligent. So why do you need protein during and after pregnancy?

The levels of protein in most woman are low due to their caloric intake. As we learned in the previous chapters, protein is loaded with amino acids that our body needs. If your body needs them when you are not pregnant, then they definitely need them when you are.

Post-baby your body is going to feel and respond differently. You just carried a baby for 9 months so that is to be expected. Not to worry though, there are a few things you can do to work your way back into a regular workout routine. Start off by making sure you are drinking lots of water and making sure you are eating a healthy diet. It's natural for mommy to be so focused on baby that she forgets about herself. Dads, make sure you take care of mom because she needs your support more than you think! Put a glass of water in front of her and help her by putting foods in her body that will fuel her. Being a mom is draining!

Remember that you have to recover so give yourself about a month or so, once you feel like you can fully bend, twist, jump, and lift weight again. Even though you feel good, you might still experience some discomfort once you start moving, so take it slow. Also, if you have had a C-section, you will need take even more precaution in your recovery. Your doctor will let you know when it's best for you to start working out and what is safest for you. In the meantime, continue to pour in proteins, vitamins, and minerals to support your recovery.

Action: Congrats Mom! You're either pregnant or going to give birth soon to a beautiful baby. Your body image may be a struggle for you but I just want you to know that you can bounce back in no time! Here are a few steps I recommend:

- Workout as much as you can while being pregnant, right up until your due date. If you experience systems of nausea, fatigue, or discomfort please stop all activity for the day.

- Find a multivitamin that sits well with you. Choose a pre-natal if pregnant, or post-natal if you've delivered. Stick with whole food prenatals.

- High quality prenatal fish oil around 600mg DHA and 120mg EPA.

- Whey protein

- Drink lots of fluids

- Write down how you feel when you work out and the times. You may or may not have to work out at the same time every day if your pregnant because the baby will learn your schedule.

- Listen to your body.

My Goals:

_____

_____

_____

_____

_____

_____

_____

CHAPTER NINE
Spiritually Fit

Our bodies are our temples. This is by far the most challenging chapter to write and in my opinion, the most important chapter of them all. Everything that I have accomplished and have the willpower to accomplish is inspired by Jesus Christ, my Lord and Savior.

A few years back I herniated my L4-L5 discs in my lower back. Moving 7 pianos a day as a piano moving specialist and fitness training had taken a toll on my body. The injury was so severe that I was put on workman's comp with no pay and my dream of a weightlifting career was over. I thought that I would be well on my way to the CrossFit regionals in no time by the way things were going, but my dreams came to a screeching halt. There I was, a young 22-year-old who could hardly walk and was suffering from the worst chronic back pain ever. My life was turned upside down and anger began to get a strong hold over me.

I continued to be ignorant and still tried to work out while making my injury increasingly worse. I was addicted to the gym, but more importantly, what others thought about me. As I shared in an earlier chapter, having been called skinny my whole life, I didn't realize how deeply that word had cut me. I just wanted to be anything other than skinny. To me, skinny equalled weak. However, that's right where I found myself. I was skinny and weak. I needed help with everything and felt fragile and small. Everything I worked so hard to achieve physically was stripped from me in the matter of a moment.

I battled with this pain for 3 years. My wife watched me go through hell and quite frankly, I don't even know how she stuck it out with me. I was such a nasty person. I saw God doing miracles in other people's lives and He even used me to bring healing in other people's bodies yet there I was, unhealed and growing bitter as a result.

If you don't have a relationship with the Lord, then some of you reading this may not understand any of what I'm saying, and you shouldn't. However, if you want to understand, you can. A personal, intimate relationship with God is a choice and I'm willing to talk with anyone who'd like to know more about that.

What I didn't know in the beginning is that the Lord wanted me to be more spiritually fit and not just physically fit. I was new in my walk and Him. He used this injury to show me many things about myself that I hadn't recognized before. He also used it to take me into a deeper relationship with Him. I had to surrender it all to Him. I had to rely *on* Him, trust *in* Him, seek *after* Him. I know While He never caused this injury, He absolutely gave me the strength I needed to endure it.

It was a constant battle. Yet despite all the anger and frustration, I had to get the Word in me (read my bible). I had to read and believe that things were going to get better simply because His Word says so! He paid the price for my healing! The bible says in Isaiah 53:5 "By His stripes we are healed (New International Version)". Today I am pain free and 100% healed! My God is awesome! If we are working out for people to notice us, to show off, and not glorify God guess what? You may get healthy but you'll never achieve true satisfaction. The bible says, "So whether you eat or drink, or whatever you do, do it all for the glory of God." (1 Corinthians 10:31 NLT) I have such a deep desire to see people set free physically, mentally, and spiritually. Not for selfish gain but for God's glory.

Rick warren said it best "Keeping your body in shape is a spiritual discipline. It's not just about losing a few pounds, wanting to live longer, or trying to look nicer."

"I urge you, brothers, in view of God's mercy, to offer your bodies as living sacrifices, holy and pleasing to God – this is your spiritual act of worship" (Romans 12:1, NIV).

I started writing this book because I heard a still small voice tell me to start writing. I believe this book is going to help those who have a true desire for change, break-thru some barriers! Honestly, I don't consider myself a writer nor do I enjoy writing, but The Holy Spirit shook me in a matter of a second and gave me the energy, motivation and determination it took to put this together for you. I'll tell you what; the look on my wife's face was priceless when I told her that I was starting to write a book. She knew it had to be God!

I understand that this health and fitness lifestyle can be the most difficult thing to get rolling. Really, I do. Is it a battle? Yes. Does it take time? Of course. Let's fight and not give up so easily! If you get hit and fall to your knees, get back up! This is your match, if you can get past the "I can't" mindset, then the battle has already been won. I can already see you rejoicing at the end of it all. The same way we trained our body to enjoy the comfort of certain foods is the same way we can train our bodies to enjoy health and fitness but we must work our muscles first! Not just physically but spiritually.

What I want to leave you with is if you want to maximize your results and quality of living you must workout, eat healthy, and supplement. If you do all three of these with consistency, you will be beyond successful. What I see too often is individuals only giving it a month and then trying something new. You need to give it time! The first month you are only getting your toes wet. You are working from the inside out. You'll will begin to see your energy increase; you will notice that you're sleeping better and that you're in an overall better mood. The second month your friends and family will start to notice the changes taking place with both your energy and your physique. It's different when other people see you because they see you differently than you see yourself and will notices changes sooner than you will. The third month you should be seeing the results yourself.

You are your worst critic because you see yourself every day. You are constantly looking in the mirror or are on the scale. That's like trying to stare at your nails and watch them as they grow out. It's crazy! I believe, now that you have these new, easy to follow tools, you are ready to successfully move forward into your health and fitness journey. Put what I have shared with you to the test and watch the results follow. One more time, the results start when you do!

Action: Are you working out for others to notice you? Are you seeking approval of others? If, so you will never be satisfied. To be set free once and for all, you must surrender and give your life to Christ. He paid it all so that you wouldn't have to carry such a heavy load. Are you ready to live a life for Christ?

He's waiting for you with open arms. What a beautiful picture. If you need someone to pray with or are looking for more information on how to move forward, please contact me. Our information is available 24/7 on our website and I would love to hear from you.

- How can you honor God with your body?
- What does romans 12:2 in the bible say?
- What does it mean that our body is a temple?

Salvation Prayer

The following is merely a guideline for your sincere step in faith. Romans 10:9 says "If you declare with your mouth, "Jesus is Lord," and believe in your heart that God raised Him from the dead, you will be saved.

"God, I recognize that I have not lived my life for You up until now. I have been living for myself and that is wrong. I need You in my life; I want You in my life. I acknowledge the completed work of Your Son Jesus Christ in giving His life for me on the cross at Calvary, and I long to receive the forgiveness you have made freely available to me through this sacrifice.

Come into my life now, Lord. Take up residence in my heart and be my king, my Lord, and my Savior. From this day forward, I will no longer be controlled by sin or the desire to please myself, but I will follow You all the days of my life. Those days are in Your hands. I ask this in Jesus' precious and holy name, Amen."

If you decided to repent of your sins and receive Christ today, welcome to God's family! Now, to grow closer to Him, the Bible tells us to follow up on our commitment.

Here are a few tips to help you along on your new journey:

- Get baptized as commanded by Christ.
- Tell someone else about your new faith in Christ.
- Spend time with God each day.
- Develop the daily habit of praying to Him and reading His Word.
- Ask God to increase your faith and your understanding of the Bible.

- Seek fellowship with other followers of Jesus. Develop a group of believing friends to answer your questions and support you.
- Find a local church where you can worship and serve.

If you have decided to follow Jesus, feel free to contact us, we would love to hear from you.

My Goals:

_____

_____

_____

_____

_____

_____

_____

REFERENCES

Association, A. D. (2016, September 19). *American Diabetes Association*. Retrieved October 1, 2016, from American Diabetes Association: www.Diabetes.org

Miller Method Episode 18 Fat Tank, Sugar Tank. *(2016)*. YouTube. *Retrieved 19 September 2016, from* https://www.youtube.com/watch?v=IVUjB921dS0

[1]National Academy of Sports Medicine. *(2016)*. Nasm.org. *Retrieved 19 September 2016, from* https://www.nasm.org/

ABOUT SHANE VEGA
Owner of VegaFit

*Crossfit Level 1 Coach

*Youth Exercise Specialist

*Elite Calisthenic Specialist

*NASM Certified Personal Trainer

*MMA Conditioning Specialist

*Performance Enhancement Specialist

*Neuromuscular Stretching

*Flexibility Training

*Positional Isometrics

*Motivational Speaker

Email: shane@vegafitelite.com

Visit us online at: vegafitelite.com

Connect with Vegafit®:

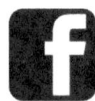

@VegaFitElite

It's time to ignite the spark of success

Everything that you need to get healthy once and for all is within you, all you need to do is tap into it.

As a professional in the health and fitness industry, I find that I am asked the same questions over and over again. People want to get results that last. They want to look and feel great. Everyone wants to end the crazy "yo-yo" cycle and experience breakthrough, yet it seems to be one of the most difficult things to do.

I believe that within these pages you'll discover the key to what you've been looking for.

This is what **BREAK-THRU** is truly all about.

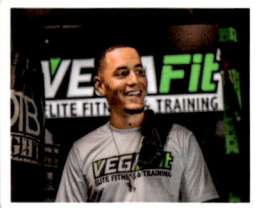

Shane Vega is founder of *Vegafit Elite Fitness & Training* located in Ewa Beach, HI. Holding 9 certifications, he is the creator of "Pain Free Sessions" that leaves clients pain free in just one session. Well known and highly sought after, Shane dedicates his life to helping people recover from a variety of pain in their bodies. Shane resides in Hawaii with his wife, Ashley and their two children Juliet & Julian.

ISBN 9781546521273

90000 >

9 781546 521273